Less Is Best

Declutter, Organize, & Simplify to Reach Minimalism; Get More Time, Money, & Energy

Original Edition

SAGE WILCOX

Less Is Best: Declutter, Organize, & Simplify to Reach Minimalism; Get More Time, Money, & Energy

First Edition, 2016

ISBN-13: 978-1-945290-09-1

ISBN-10: 1-945290-09-9

Library of Congress Control Number: 2016955756

Printed in the United States of America.

DEDICATION/ACKNOWLEDGMENTS

This is dedicated to all of the people who are working hard to simplify their lives and better their situations, day by day, and in every way. Perseverance and discipline pays off. YOU deserve to make your dreams come true and reach your full potential, and this book is for you. Enjoy!
Deep, humble appreciation to the Divine Source, whom I aspire to grow closer to every day, in faith.

Thanks to all who made this book possible. Also to those who loved and supported me as I worked on getting it published. You know who you are, and I am so appreciative and grateful.

And last but not least, to the readers. Thank you for taking the time to read this book. I hope you enjoy it and find something inside that resonates and inspires you in some way. Thank you. Let's pour our favorite drink, find a comfortable spot, and get started, shall we? Our dreams and goals are waiting to be fulfilled.

Other books by Sage Wilcox:

- *Love Letters from Exes: Proof That Life Goes On After a Break Up and Love Is What You Make It*
- *Get It Up: 101 Ways to Raise Your Vibration, Reduce Stress, Depression, & Anxiety, Increase Joy, Peace, & Happiness and Attract Abundance Automatically!*
- *The 2-Hour Vacation: Let Go and Relax, Reduce Stress & Anxiety, Gain Inner Peace, and Happiness*
- *Until We Fall (A Romance Novel)*
- *The Importance of Doing It: How to Utilize Discipline to Get Out of Bed, and Make Your Dreams Come True! A Guide to Taking Action to Create Successful Habits, Reduce Stress, Anxiety, & Depression & Gain Self-Discipline, Motivation, & Success!*

Please visit her website at:
http://sagewilcox.wix.com/books

CONTENTS

PREFACE

"The secret of happiness, you see, is not found in seeking more, but in developing the capacity to enjoy less."
~ Socrates

You didn't pick this book up by accident. If there is something stirring inside of you that is drawing you towards minimalism, then go for it! The key is in the action, though. You can read this book over and over, but if you don't take action, nothing will happen and you won't reach your goals. Make a list of your why's right now, and then take action. Remember to be patient with yourself, but not too patient. You want to see progress. You want to see results, and you will!

I like to include testimonies from real people in my books because I believe it is through other people's stories that we can relate and learn. We can see that many others have done it and are reaping the benefits and rewards that come from the minimalist lifestyle.

The call to lead a minimalist lifestyle is one that comes from deep within each person. For me, I am grateful that the call came to me when it did. I have noticed that in the last decade the call is becoming more frequent among a larger swath of society, as more of the general population strays further from what is important towards what is profitable. In the process of doing that, we have laid to waste everything from our mind to our planet, and we have silenced whatever remnants of greatness we may have been building up to as a species.

Minimalism is an unfortunate misnomer, but necessary to drive the point home that what we have chosen to prioritize; many of these things have steered our ship in the wrong direction. But this can be changed. And we don't need to change it because we want to change the world. We need to make this change so that we can embrace the abundance that the universe offers us. But we have traded our appreciation for that which is abundant and good for that which is worthless. In the process, we have sacrificed the invaluable for that which has no value.

Whichever direction our ship has been sailing, the rudder that can guide us back on course is our mindset. If we embrace the right mindset, the change that is needed occurs with little discomfort or the need to exert excessive energy.

Life is actually quite easy; it is the complications of going after things we don't need, using resources we don't have, to satisfy the definition of greatness by someone we don't know that throws a wrench into the entire system.

Our greatest asset is our mind and the consciousness that lies deep within. But if you bury those powerful tools under the cloud of distractions, they tend to lay there in waste. You have to make the conscious decision to clear the clutter and allow your inner self to shine through.

Most of what steers us off course are distractions. These distractions are in our control so long as we identify them and know what we are capable of. You are capable of more than you give yourself credit for.

It is in becoming aware, that we are able to grow and move forward to who we truly are meant to be. Becoming aware of distractions that do not serve us, and of false belief systems that we have seemingly picked up along the way by others, is the first step.

We see distractions everywhere and think that they are external, but that's not always the case. For some, alcohol is a distraction, for others, it's not. If something is a distraction for one, shouldn't it be a distraction for everyone? But man's vice can be another man's virtue. The key is for you to locate your own distractions. The problem with distractions, is that their very nature precludes you from identifying them until you return your life to living with only what you need - the life of a minimalist.

The human consciousness is simple in its complexity; clear in its irony; strong in its weakness; and, brave in its fear. As such, when we challenge the lazy, unmotivated, cluttered view of all things that encapsulate our world we find that our reality - what may seem real to us, is not reality at all. Which is why when we hear something as ironic as less is best, we recoil in its apparent stupidity; or in its genius, depending on where we are on the arc of enlightenment.

I am an apostate of materialism who once worshiped at the altar of wealth, poured libations at the temple of desire, and bore witness to the religion of greed. Then one day, I gave it all up. All of my necessities now fits into a large backpack and I am richer than I have ever been at any other point in my life.

As we journey through the course of this book I will share with you my personal experience about this decision and how it played out during the transition. It has been six years since that day and the consequences of my actions have exceeded my expectations.

Let's be clear about one thing. I did not give up everything so that my life will be spent in search of the illusory truth. I did not give up everything so that I could chill and hang out. And, I certainly did not do it because I wanted to experience poverty. On the contrary, I gave everything up so that I could experience richness.

That's the irony of life.
Throughout the experience of letting go, which came in stages, oscillating between the release of mental baggage,

and physical baggage, the result was an increase in clarity of all things that mattered and of all things that could be accomplished with less baggage.

As we continued to unload we started to see that other things would come into our lives, and as those things came we would consider holding on to it because it felt like in not doing so we would be sweeping away blessings that came our way. It was amazing how the prospect of new stuff would attempt to derail our resolve to live simply.

When we got over it and gave that away, we found that even more opportunities came our way. It was as though the more we decided we didn't want things, the more life sent us better things. But we continuously gave those away too. In the midst of going through multiple cycles of this, we started to experience a new reality. It was the reality of true freedom. When you are beholden to nothing, you are truly free, and that freedom brings with it a new form of clarity. Some would say that this new form of clarity brings you to the face of God, or closer to the Divine Source/Creator.

Whatever you believe minimalism in all reality, is a moving experience. The face of God we speak of is not like the Shroud of Turin or a physical face, it's a metaphor to describe the level of purity that we felt in the freedom that was the result of simplicity when severing our connection to materialism.

When we converted to living the life of minimalists, a number of effects reverberated through our family. From understanding the true nature of joy and happiness to being able to identify the realities of life and the abundant opportunities around us. We also started to see the power of faith and the amazing wonder and awe of all things that we were experiencing in our everyday lives.

Come along. Your freedom awaits.

CHAPTER 1
THE ESSENTIAL MINDSET

"We make a living by what we get, we make a life by what we give."
~ Sir Winston Churchill

The most powerful mind, the fastest wit, the strongest muscles do not amount to much if the person has a severe lack of clarity. Operating under a cloud is a debilitating curse and it is a situation that afflicts most of us. That brain fog, that we sometimes get, trips us up as we charge for the finish line and knocks us off our feet as we jump for the stars. This cloud feels no different from a brain fog that you get under the auspices of a severe hangover, but there is no physical toxin at play here. Just the intoxication of greed. In line with this, is the all too familiar wanting what we don't have syndrome. Or the grass is greener on the other side.

In the wake of the eighties' Oliver Stone movie, Wall Street the phrase "greed is good" shot to prominence. It seemed like a good mantra at the time, and it still does for many people. The essential mindset of those in this crowd is one that gives prominence to a part of us that subscribes to the view that wealth is limited.

The irony here is that they profess the belief in the abundance of the universe but then display the actions of greed like there isn't enough of what they are going for to go around. That's the first inconsistency. If you believe in an abundant universe, and the power of attraction, you cannot believe in hoarding.

"To live a pure unselfish life, one must count nothing as one's own in the midst of abundance."
~Buddha

Greed/want is the prevailing mindset that exists in those who subscribe to the essential economic model of capitalism. It is misconceived by proponents and detractors alike, that capitalism is greed and hoarding. It is not. Capitalism is about the ownership of goods by the people and everyone gets paid for what they work for and what they risk. Capitalism still works within the context of need vs greed. Except in giving and relinquishing the small stuff, we empty our cup and make room for the big stuff.

There is something mysterious that happens when you give up the greed and the insecurity that comes with it. To label it as miraculous will diminish its value within some crowds while piquing the interest of others. But, I am going to stay away from whitewashing this with the shade of religion.

There were lots of examples in my life that I will point to as we traverse the pages of this book. The first one that comes to mind is the mindset that inevitably comes with not letting go.

During my working life as a successful banker, I made sure that I had the best insurance policy I could to protect my family. It sounds like the right thing to do, if one can afford it, right? For the 18 years that I've had my policy, I cannot remember a year that I have not used it at least four times in any given year. When we gave up everything, it included our insurance. In the last six years since we made the move, not once has a situation arisen that we have had the need to rely on that policy.

We also gave up our credit cards, and guess what? Not once, since we gave credit cards up, did we find the need to use them. When we had them, there was always something that we needed to buy, something that we needed to have or something emergent. All that stopped after we cut the cards up.

The last time we were at a mall, aimlessly touring its many shops in search of something to buy, was more than five years ago.

As humans we are at the mercy of our mindset. The bad thing is that we can get swept away in its ferocity. The good thing is that we can take control of it. The best environment for a healthy mindset is when the mind is clear.

Clarity comes in many forms, the main tenet of clarity is the lack of distraction and the preponderance of focus. There is a certain gravity in being when you have none of these distractions to skew your focus.

CHAPTER 2
CLEARING OUT THE CLUTTER

"Any half-awake materialist well knows – that which you hold onto holds you."
~ Tom Robbins

It takes a certain kind of skill to make a list of the clutter that you are going to discard. Because the first challenge is in identifying all the things that are clutter in nature. The secret is that you will come to find out one day that it is all clutter.

If you have three sets of summer clothes, one of it is clutter, because you only need two. If you have two copies of Treasure Island in your library, both of them are clutter. Well, that's only possible in today's environment, because we have immediate access via the internet now, not to mention we have access to our town library as well.

When my family and I got rid of everything, it even included our library of books which I had collected over the course of my life and then merged it with my spouse's collection when we got married. As the children came along their books piled on top of ours. Every single one of them is gone, even the ones signed by the authors. Instead, we have electronic copies that reside in the cloud, accessible at any point we are in the mood to read our favorite passage or chapter.

The clutter is gone, but the wealth remains.

There are two kinds of clutter. One is the physical clutter that you see about you. You will be surprised to realize, in your own time, that most of what you won, most of your possessions, whether purchased, or gifted, or inherited actually have little use in your daily life.

Look around you where you sit right now, what objects come into your view? When you get done reading this chapter, or if you'd like to pause here, that's fine too, go ahead and make a list of every item that the eye can see from where you stand (or sit) and make a list of it. Once you have a list mark each one with a 'Y' or an 'N'. Y for Yes, you need it and you can't live without it. If you lost it, you couldn't go on. The N on the list is placed next to the items that you know for a certain fact that even if you were to get up and get rid of it this minute, you would not miss it in a day, two days, or even a decade. You could live without it.

When I made that list, guess what happened? There was a N next to every item that was in my study. (That's where I made the list.) Of course, you need not visit my study to realize that marking Y next to every single item wouldn't be realistic. Certainly, there must have been something that made the cut? Something that had to go? No, on my very first list nothing made the cut. I felt as though I needed all of it.

A few days later it occurred to me how absurd that was. Seemingly out of nowhere did I feel anchored to every one of these items that I had absolutely felt certain that I could not live without.

It turns out, our possessions are not really our possessions. We don't possess them, they possess us and we are enslaved to them. That realization made me sick to my stomach because suddenly it dawned on me how enslaved I really was. When we moved to this house, one of our biggest considerations was that we needed space for all the stuff we had. Most of the real estate we lived in was not there to shield us from the elements. It was there to house our possessions. Think about the money we spend buying the house, the loan costs, the interest on that loan, the maintenance, and all that goes along with it, so that we could keep a bunch of things which we hardly visited once a year.

Even if you put aside all the monetary considerations and file it away under the heading of "not everything's about money". I am still left with one glaring fact, that upon inspection, doing all of that made absolutely no sense.

It turns out, your possessions are a validation of your ego. Those inanimate objects that you hardly use are a validation to your ego. What's more is that when you made the purchase of that item, you had to have, most likely it was done for reasons other than utility.

"Too many people spend money they haven't earned, to buy things they don't want, to impress people they don't like."
~ Will Rogers

Let me give you another example. The first bed and mattress I purchase after moving out on my own, and when I had a job, was fairly comfortable. When it grew tired, I replaced it with something a little more expensive and the afternoon it arrived I was feeling pretty good about myself in that I was able to afford a slightly more expensive mattress. I imagined how much better my sleep would be. The first few nights were great but after the second week, I started experiencing back pain.

I endured for a few months and after the advice of some all-knowing friends, I replaced that mattress. It was significantly more expensive, look fabulous and promised a healthier back.

A few weeks later the aches returned. A year later the mattress was replaced. This happened a total of four times, each time the mattress and its accessories escalated in price. When we moved, that mattress came with us and my backache, now bordering on chronic, followed as well.

The doctors had all kinds of advice. And as long as my insurance was covering it, the inconvenience was minimal.

The night we emptied the house I went to sleep on my straw mat with a bruised ego from not having any possessions, and a sore back. The morning after, I woke up on my new straw mat, with an unfamiliar feeling. Well, a number of unfamiliar feelings. First off, when I opened my eyes, was the fact that I was two feet lower in altitude and the ceiling was a lot further away than I had remembered. The second thing was that I had not woken up during the night and apparently had a full night's rest - something that I had not experienced in a while. But most amazing to me was that I had zero back pain. Zero.

I won't go through every instance of my cleansing, as I call it, but I will say that every time I released something, I got a lot more peace than I thought I would get. More than I could've imagined. Like in the case of the mattress, each time I purchased a more expensive mattress I thought I was buying better sleep, better posture, and back health, and I was certainly feeding my ego with the knowledge that

I could afford to spend a large sum of money on a mere mattress. But upon relinquishing it, I received peace and health, which, individually are amazing gifts, but together, are miracles. Bertrand Russell, the philosopher was correct when he said, "It is preoccupation with possession, more than anything else, that prevents men from living freely and nobly."

So start by evaluating each room. Some people like to gather all of their clothes into one pile, or books, or mementos, etc. But I have found going room by room can be just as effective, if not easier. I have also found that going room by room helps to motivate people to keep going with less chance of becoming overwhelmed. Once one room is done, you start to see real results., and rather quickly. It is an amazing feeling. Scan each room. At first, you will notice many things that you obviously don't need. The start of this process is by far the easiest. Look around, gather the obvious items that you can get rid of and either box or bag them up to donate or throw away. Once all of the obvious things are out of the way, you will need to start getting specific by going shelf by shelf, draw by draw , or hanger by hanger. Try not to take too long on each item; this is where a lot of people get hung up and get discouraged. Remember you are not your things and they do not define you. You should not keep an item unless it makes you feel good deep down inside. I have one client who had two lamps stored in the far end of his barn where he rarely every saw them. His grandmother had made them out of seashells while she was alive. They were very large and had been sitting in the back of the garage for over 16 years. They looked very dirty, dusty, and weathered. My client couldn't bear to part with them because his grandmother had made them, but he didn't want them inside his home either. I asked him how they made him feel. How did he feel when he came upon them in the back of his barn? He said he felt sad and guilty when he looked at them. He felt like he should use them but they just wouldn't fit in his small home. I asked my client if he wanted to leave them for his two sons. He laughed and expressed that he knew without a doubt that his two sons would not want them. “So what are you holding onto them for?” They obviously didn’t bring him joy and happiness. “Do you think you will miss them if they are gone?” I asked. He knew that he wouldn’t. This is just one example of how and why we hold onto things.

Go room by room, evaluating and defining what you *need.* In my experience you will need to do this over and over until it becomes second nature. Minimalism is an adjustment and it takes practice. But it’s well worth it. Some people can do this and get it done successfully in just a few weeks, becoming true minimalists. I have found, however, that the vast majority of people need approximately 6 months or so. They go room by room and then repeat, finding more things that they do not need. I like to tell my clients to start in the bathroom, as this is a room that tends to be the less cluttered. Clean out and get rid of old shampoo bottles, get rid of candles, décor, and clutter that you don’t need. We are going for minimalism We are retraining our brains. Less is best. Once the bathroom is done, move onto a bedroom, den, or closet. Once every room is done, repeat. Each time you will find more that you can get rid of. Do this until you are satisfied.

Be sure that you are continually reading books, blogs, articles, etc. on the subject of minimalism. Books on minimalism will help you see the truth and help change your mindset We need to break the deformative programming that has been done by advertisers and the like. Reading informative articles on minimalism will motivate you and give you additional ideas to keep up with your minimalist lifestyle. It is very easy, in this world that we live in, to get distracted and to head down the wrong path and back towards our old habits. You will be bombarded with distractions and by people who don’t understand, but minimalism offers true freedom, and you recognize that. Read on about profiling distractions

CHAPTER 3
PROFILING DISTRACTIONS

"One way to boost our willpower and focus is to manage our distractions instead of letting them manage us."
~Daniel Goleman

There are many kinds of distractions. Some distractions are caused by others, and some we bring upon ourselves. But most distractions are in our control. If focus is a state of being that we invoke, then distractions are the antithesis of that focus - they are essentially different sides of the same coin. Logically then, if the focus is ours, then the distraction is ours also.

Distractions have become so prevalent that we have been programmed to not have the patience to sit still for more than 30 seconds. We can't sit at a stoplight without checking our phones. Heck, some of us can't even drive without checking it. Thankfully, driving and phone usage is illegal, as it should be, but I can't begin to tell you how many people I see looking at their phones while driving. It's as bad as drinking and driving, in my opinion, but that's beside the point. My point is that we have learned that distractions are normal and that in fact we don't know what to do without them. Freedom lies in being free from distractions no matter what is going on around you, or what is tempting you to succumb to it. We need to start training and telling our minds what to do. Meditation can help with this. We are not our minds or our bodies. And we can learn to use both to our advantage once we train them correctly. It's so exciting! We can train our minds so that it will listen. But it takes persistence, practice, and discipline. Your mind is used to doing what it wants. Eating what it wants, buying what it wants, thinking about what it wants. Once you learn to master distractions, you will be able to master all other areas of your life.

The main strain of distraction, its DNA, is the nature of its existence. That nature is in our heads. Distractions are not tangible in and of themselves. Certainly. A TV is a tangible item, so is an XBox, but the ability to get derailed from finishing a term paper because one hears the paddles of the controller beckoning does not make the XBox culpable in our distraction.

Distractions are intangible in their nature no matter how tangible they are in space and time.

Since distractions are intangible, then we need an intangible force to counter them and that force has been long assumed to be the force of will. Willpower is indeed a force, but there is a better, less brutish alternative. That alternative is the graceful decision to sidestep the distraction before it manifests.

Habit is also a distraction, and the more one vanquishes his habits, the lesser the distractions that will vex him.

Removing possessions are a higher form of distraction dilution. A lot of what you possess creates a significant distraction, taking away from your time, your energy and more importantly taking away from your potential to achieve greater heights of peace and true prosperity and abundance.

There is one thing that is worth pointing out at this juncture and that is that distractions prevent you from being all that your potential says you can be. Distractions are rooted in things that you don't need, and those things that you don't need are in no way the riches you've been told they are.

Up to this point, most people have been duped into thinking that possessions are richness. Possessions may symbolize richness, but they are not richness in and of themselves.

Commercialization and profits have resulted in sophisticated strategies and methods to tap into the psychology of people and sell them things they don't need. To be more precise, advertisers make their pitch directly to the ego and define the path that the ego should take.

The gratification that comes from falling for the advertising message creates a self-fulfilling prophecy and that creates value in the product. All the while, that product is merely a symbol of the richness that people desire and deserve.

The human mind, the human consciousness are powerful forces that can ask and receive almost anything we wish for because the universe provides. But the condition of the power is that it must be done with clarity.

CHAPTER 4
SIMPLIFY

"Make things as simple as possible but no simpler."
~ Albert Einstein

When you have clutter, it is hard to simplify. When you can't simplify, whatever is in excess is a cause for distraction. Distraction takes you off your path for peace and the lake of peace clouds your daily existence.

When you see the wisdom in simplification, you will be able to see that all great things are no more complex than they need to be. Look at the most powerful invention in the history of the world - the wheel. Look at the power of this invention, and compare it to the simplicity of its design.

Our mind is the same way. It is the most powerful when it is the simplest. Simple is not the same as inadequate. Some of the most compelling logic that the mind can make is also the simplest of all.

Take for instance some of the most lethal viruses or highly dangerous bacteria. They are difficult to annihilate but their structure is one of the simplest. The problem with the human culture is that we associate simple with ineffective or puerile. We associate simple with lack, when really simple means uncomplicated, easy, and presenting no difficulty. Life does not have to be difficult. It can be simple and easy, free from chaos, confusion, and worry.

Learning to Let it Go

When you make the decision to live a life of simplicity, you are forced to learn a valuable lesson - the ability to let things go. At the bottom of it all, is the mental affinity, or the psychological affection that you develop with things. This is a misplaced notion that you will need to learn to let go of.

We are all born with this because it is the initial instinct that keeps us close to our parents and our responsibility is to hold on. One of the early physical abilities of a child is the ability to hold on with both hands, and you witness that when a baby holds on to his mother. That notion of holding on is a safety mechanism so that he doesn't fall or get separated from a parent.

The thing that keeps us safe is also one that causes us a tremendous amount of headaches in the older years of our lives. And therein lies the lesson we can take with us across a number of other areas in our lives as well. The lesson is this: all the habits that we carry with us from childhood to adult life is one that is mostly inappropriate from one stage in our life to the next stage. It is up to us to consciously move our habits from one stage to the next. It is not just the habits of childhood that force its way into our adult life, it is also the habits of our adulthood that flow from a younger stage to an older one.

Take for instance the desire to remain attractive to the

opposite sex. If you think about it, that desire to remain attractive to the opposite sex should only be in service during the period that is optimal for childbearing. But because we can't seem to let go, because it's a habit with a high payoff, we find it extremely difficult to let go. We hold on to our youth and fear the aging process. We hold on to vanity and pride, and in so doing we complicate our lives and miss out on tremendous peace, acceptance, and joy.

Not letting go is one of the most profound causes of complications that we can easily avoid. Because it is not just an issue of vanity. The issue pervades a number of other areas as well and becomes highly complex for us to weed out. Think about a woman's hesitancy to reveal her age. Where do you think that comes from? It is rooted in her inability to let go.

"The greatest step towards a life of simplicity is to learn to let go."
~ Steve Maraboli

Learning to let go is a two-part exercise. And knowing what to let go is one of the main cogs in achieving a life that is full and satisfying.

To get started, there are two major parts of letting go that you will need to work out. The first is that of physical objects that you need to let go of in your life. The second involves the non-physical areas of your life that you need to let go. The interesting thing about them is that they work in lockstep. They are closely related and work together.

You will go through stages where you let go of intangible fragments in your life and that will help unlock parts of you that will release physical objects in your life, and that will in turn swing back to intangible fragments in your mind.

This is a major step and period in your life when you do this. For women, especially when they reach the age of menopause, it is an excellent opportunity to purge the system of tangible and intangible items that will help them be a lot freer and happier when they come out the other side. Unfortunately, society teaches us tips and tricks on how to hold on even harder and that becomes a problem for the individual and for all of those around them as well. This is an example of learned behavior that does not benefit us. And if we are not careful, we will teach this, unknowingly, to our children and future generations without even giving it much thought. Here is where deliberate action is needed. The action of becoming aware.

Trying Harder

This is one of the hardest decision to make if you are clouded, and one of the easiest to make when you are clear. That's why less is always best because it gives you clarity of what to let go of and of what to keep.

"Letting go or to try harder is one of the hardest decision you will ever make."
Anonymous

At every juncture of the letting go stage you will have a sense of doubt over what you can and should let go or what you should hold on to and try harder at. But the choice is rather simple and it is something I spent a lot of effort and energy learning. It can be confusing when you are clouded, but the best way to make the difference is to look at the impetus to let go.

Here is how you decide. If you are trying to achieve something, and it's hard, that voice that you hear in the back of your head to let it go, is the voice of doubt, confusion, and failure. Never listen to that. When you let go, it has to be on your terms not because someone or something is asking you to give up, but because you know, on a spiritual level, that it needs to be done. Letting go is never the same as giving up. Letting go is good for your soul, giving up or quitting is detrimental to your being. There is a big difference.

When you attempt something, nothing should ever convince you to let it go. Achieving something can come at a great personal sacrifice and there is a lot that we should learn to let go, but do not let go of the objective and the effort to move forward. This is the point where you try harder. This is the point where you shake it off, get up, dust yourself off and invoke the clarity you need to get it done.

Simplicity and Letting Go

What does all this trying harder and letting go have to do with simplifying your life? Because simplifying your life involves letting go, and letting go allows you to be clear enough to let go even more. Once you start to really grasp this, the letting go will begin to flow effortlessly in all areas of your life.

Letting go comes in stages, you can't let go of everything all at once, and even when you think you have let go of everything, there will be areas which you will learn still need to be let go of as well. For me letting go of expensive possessions was comparatively easy and letting go of mementos was hard. So the material stuff got tossed first and as I cleaned mental house, my new uncluttered life made it easier to see that mementos were just another form of holding on.

I know people who keep old McDonald toys and find it very hard to throw them away. I recently helped someone clean house after the death of her husband. This was during a time where I thought that I had fully let go of everything in my life. But to silently look at this person's life, I found that there are many people who just cannot bring themselves to get rid of anything. In this particular case, this person had accumulated so many things over 70 years of his life that we did not even know where to begin.

In the end, we managed to get rid of only 10% of it before the spouse was in tears and could not let go of the other 90% because she was convinced it was a betrayal of her husband's memories.

So we stopped. A year later we tried again and managed to get rid of a few more things. This went on for five years. And there was still plenty of things left to go. But by this point, she had more peace about his death. She was less burdened, and she had a slight bounce to her step that had not been there before.

The sixth year was the charm where we managed to get rid of all the things that were left over. All of it was donated to various shelters and homes for the elderly. Over the course of two weeks of solid work, we cleared their home of everything that didn't need to be there.

When she finally let go of all those things and the memory (and grief) attached to some of those things, instead of forgetting her husband, there was a change in her. The memoirs were no longer external and vexing, they had become part of her and they were a cause of joy instead of a cause of pain. She had somehow transformed into a person who was richer from the experience, than a person burdened by loss. The transformation from letting go was nothing short of a miracle, and she said she wished she would have, and could have done it sooner.

When we came home from that trip we found the clarity to unload more even more of our things, this time in terms of unnecessary memories and useless mementos.

The funny thing was that we were trying to teach this wonderful person the promise of letting go, and in the end, we learned more just by watching her transformation. She was freer, lighter, and happier. It motivated us to keep moving forward and to keep simplifying our own lives.

CHAPTER 5
WHY MORE IS ATTRACTIVE

"You have succeeded in life when all you really want is only what you really need."
~ Vernon Howard

Let's pause for a minute on the path to simplification and ask ourselves: Why is the concept of more so attractive? As you ponder this question, let me offer you one more dimension that will help you in answering the question.

The idea of more is something that most people don't understand and is often taken for granted, yet we get tongue-tied when the question is posed. Why is the concept of more so attractive? It seems like one of those questions where the truth seems self-evident, but it's not. The concept of more is rooted in the way the body works and the way it has evolved over time. It's a question of economics and survival - sort of the 'economics of survival'.

Economics of Survival

At the core of the desire for more is the concept of storage for a rainy day. You see squirrels do this, and it works really well for them. You see camels do this as well and it works out for them as well. Because these animals believe that the possibility of gaining food at a certain point in the future (in the case of the camel it's water that they are worried about - and so they store it in their humps). So this mechanism is built into us deep down into the core of our primitive brain. The two fundamental purposes of the human body are contained in the brain stem. This is the area of the entire brain that is primitive. It is called primitive because it is the oldest in the series of development in the brainstem, and it is also in control of our primitive instincts which include self-preservation and species preservation - in other words, sex.

In the economics of survival, there is always an inherent risk of the next meal not being there. Depending on how high you are on the food chain, one of the ways of overcoming the possibility of starving is to be able to hoard food. Hoarding becomes extremely important to the body as the act of holding on. Holding on and hoarding are both tied to the prime instinct of the human body.

It is also a biological fact that when a body is subjected to hunger, even once, or over the course of time, where the intake of food is insufficient, the body changes its metabolism to convert more of the food intake into storage than to use up the food as energy. Laziness may kick in as a form of energy conversion and conservation.

The body's mechanism is designed to be able to store food for a time when there is nothing to eat. The logic algorithm here is automated and happens somewhere in the basic instinct of the body - the primitive brain. The same goes for nursing the young, when a mother first gives birth, one of the triggers of the milk to let down, is the sound of a baby's cry. If the mother has a lack of food, then whatever food intake she does receive goes first towards basic systems and then towards the production of milk for the child. The point here is that the body is built from a physical and primitive level to hoard in case of emergencies.

The body runs on a very different set of systems than the mind. In fact, at some points in time the body and mind can come up in opposition against one another. The systems of the body are controlled by the loudest parts of the central nervous system and the higher functions of the brain, which developed later in the evolutionary process, are in the new parts of the brain in the cerebrum and cerebellum.

One of the ways that the lower part of the brain convinces the higher part of the brain is that it floods the brain with pleasure hormones. Take for instance Dopamine, which is made and stored in the hypothalamus. Dopamine is located in one of the oldest parts of the brain and released in the prefrontal cortex as part of the reward mechanism. Dopamine is not the only pleasure hormone, there are others.

The bottom line is that whenever one takes on more things, the brain is rewarded by the flood of dopamine. Although in smaller quantities than it is rewarded by sex and food, nonetheless, it becomes habit forming and we learn, by this dopamine release, to search for more and to hoard more. We even take more of anything we can get our hands on because the brain is being rewarded each time we take more of something. It doesn't even matter what it is. Look at a person's behavior at a buffet line. We hoard but don't necessarily consume. And when we consume, we don't necessarily need it, and we end up over eating. And so the wheels turn and we can see how this mechanism can result in addictive habits.

Just as we can be addicted to substances like tobacco, alcohol, and drugs, or to actions like sex, or even to negative thoughts, it is not a simple matter of deciding to do or not to do, there are larger forces at play.

To avoid these forms of addiction, a simple life, where we find the happiness that less clutter brings, helps to overcome negative habits and the negative effects that become central to our lives when blocked by clutter and complications.

The rushing of hormones to promote one thing or the other complicates the way we behave and detracts from what we can accomplish. We go from being infants that cling to our parents for everything, then we outgrow that in the pubescent years only to morph into young adults, middle-aged adults after that, and then we move into our wiser senior years. Each stage of our life is designed to work (and learn) from experience from the earlier stage, but not designed to mimic that stage.

When the primitive brain rewards the higher brain for things that it thinks it needs, it forms a habit in that part of the brain, so much so, that once the primitive side has moved on, the higher brain is caught in the world wind of habits that it thinks it needs to accomplish. And often times it finds that the reward is no longer there. This can sometimes lead to depression.

Menopause and midlife crisis are typically times when these manifest.

More is Not Always the Answer

As we grow older and the purpose for our lives differs, we find that hoarding is a way of clinging to the past, and while it may bring temporary relief to the pain and fear of change, it is actually accumulating long-term grief. The best way to overcome this is to embrace and appreciate the present moment. First one minute at a time, then one day at a time, and then one year at a time. But most importantly, we need to embrace each moment, which is not really the measure of time, but rather the measure of our place in life. All we have is now.

Not only is more not always the answer, it seems to be true that more is never the answer especially when it is fueled by uncertainty.

Faith

Faith is something you hear a lot about in religious and spiritual circles, and sometimes it has come to mean something very different from what it really is. Before we get into what it really is, you must know that the way to counter the desire for more, is by having faith.

Faith is a product of the higher mind functions. It is hard to invoke faith when you are diving into the base areas of the brain where you are driven by primal instincts. If you have faith that the next meal will present itself when the time is right, then when you are presented with the current meal, you are going to react exactly by what you need and not more.

Faith is like a coin. It has two sides to it. It has a physical side and an intangible side. The tangible side consists of your actions and the intangible side consists of your feelings. Both are severely misunderstood.

Faith is not the belief of something that you cannot empirically prove (it can be that, but it's not all that). We only get half the picture when we see that faith is believing in something blindly while hoping that it shows up.

The first thing we need to do is realize that not everything that happens in our life happens within detection of our five senses. Not everything can be seen, heard, tasted, smelt or felt. And when you believe something is present, even though it cannot show itself to you (because you are limited by your five senses), then this is called faith.

This opens you up to a lot of mischief that can be perpetrated upon you. Faith is all the things that you cannot detect by your senses, but it is detectable by your mind. If you reflect on something long enough, you can see it for what it is and you can detect and attach to its veracity and truth.

That's the first half of faith.

The second half of faith is that you act in promotion of what your mind believes is present. This is the tangible side of the equation. When you act in certainty of something you believe in, you are not afraid that it will manifest. You know that it will.

Most people who hoard either have no faith, or have a very misguided view of faith, or have only partial faith because they seem to always miss out the tangible side of faith.

When you combine both sides of faith with clarity of vision, what you end up with is a very powerful force you can use to accomplish almost anything.

Do you know one of the main reasons Augustus Caesar was one of the most successful of all Roman Emperors and served successfully as emperor for 40 years, after converting Rome from a Republic, was how he lived? One of his most powerful weapons was that he, amidst all his wealth and power, lived the life of a minimalist.

By living the life of a minimalist, Augustus displayed the single most powerful quality of any successful person and that is the quality of faith. This faith fed into the clarity that was needed to rule and accomplish feats unthinkable by those who are clouded and weighed down by things.

CHAPTER 6
PROFILE OF A MINIMALIST

"Have nothing in your homes that you do not know to be useful or believe to be beautiful."
~ William Morris

Augustus Caesar, whom we mentioned in the last chapter was Rome's first emperor who served for forty years, without the need to force people to support him. In fact, the people begged him to become emperor. Instead of sleeping in luxury, he slipped on a woven mat and ate simple cheese and fruit for his meals.

Not only was he one of the richest and wealthiest men in the world at the time, he was also a minimalist who did not seek to spend his wealth. He remained a minimalist for most of his life.

Many rich and famous celebrities have chosen the minimalist lifestyle because of the freedom that lies within it. As well as past gurus and saints. Jesus, Buddha, Mother Teresa, to name just a few.

Here are ten steps for you to ramp up your achievement levels by becoming a minimalist like Augustus. This may seem extreme at first, but these are the steps to achieving the freedom (financially, spiritually, and emotionally) that comes from becoming a minimalist.

I recently was told about a blog a woman had written on how she only wore the same thing for over a year. She had three pairs of pants that were identical and three shirts that were identical. She said she had so much freedom and a lot more time because of this one simple change she had made in her life. Again, for many, this will seem extreme, but trust me, if you are serious about wanting more (of everything) this is the way to go.

Ten Steps to Being a Minimalist

1. Own three sets of clothes. One to wear, while one is being washed, and the other as a change to freshen up. Make sure each is identical so that you do not spend time on deciding what to wear on a given day. When you wear the same clothes, you lose vanity and save time. Donate the rest of your clothes.
2. Discard things you don't use. From books, you don't read, to plates you store in the attic. If you don't use it often, you don't need it.
3. Buy a travel bag that you can carry on your back, and place all that you need in the bag. If it doesn't fit, you don't need it.
4. If you have a large home, sell it and buy one that is smaller and more efficient for you and your family. You don't need a two car garage, an attic, a basement, five guestrooms, three bathrooms, and so on. All you need is a place to shelter you from the elements.
5. Eat what you need. Train yourself to eat what is necessary and not what is extravagant.

6. Walk more often. Reduce your dependence on a personal car. Sell your car(s) and walk, take public transport, use a bicycle if you have to and take trains or buses when traveling in the city or long distances. It is the best way for you to absorb nature and to keep yourself healthy.
7. Plant some or all of your food. Make as much of your food as practicable.
8. Convert all your documents and books to electronic format and keep them in the cloud.
9. Keep one day a week to rest, reflect, meditate, and reconnect with nature. Observe silence on this day.
10. Get rid of your TV. Commercials are the worst thing you can subject yourself to and so are most of the typical programming which are a drain on your mind and your strength. Commercial advertising is the opposite of being a minimalist and it is the antithesis of clarity.

Not everyone is ready to do all of these right away. It took me four years to really accomplish most of what is on the list, and I am still working on it. We even sold our desktop computers and shrunk our electronic footprint down to laptops and tablets. We moved everything to the cloud for the purpose of being able to travel light and live light.

One of the immediate effects we noticed was that we found we had no more worry. We no longer cared about break-ins when we were not home. We didn't worry about losing anything because we no longer owned anything worth stealing. Even if our devices were stolen or lost, the data would still be available to us, we would just have to replace the device. All these actions brought us freedom. We no longer worried. Only one person disliked all we did - our insurance agent, who lost a sizeable chunk of commission when we canceled our life insurance, our auto insurance because we no longer had a vehicle, and we chose the lowest health insurance plan necessary.

We didn't realize how much we spent trying to protect

stuff we had already spent money on.

From all the walking we do, all the healthy food we eat, all the excesses we don't consume, not only have we found happiness, we have found health in ourselves, joy in our families, and achievement of our objectives.

The life of a minimalist has brought us more than we ever anticipated living the life of materialism.

CHAPTER 7
LESSONS FROM A MINIMALIST

"Minimalism is not subtraction for the sake of subtractions; Minimalism is the subtraction for the sake of focus."
~ Unknown

Some people embrace minimalism to get in touch with humility. Some do it because it feels noble. Others do it because becoming rich and working in today's world can get complicated. But, as a person who has done it, who started out with one reason, and continued for a different one, I can tell you that being a minimalist is about gaining the world.

I am no biblical scholar, by any means, but there are a number of passages in the New Testament, some for the Koran, even the Torah and the Gita, that come up and jolt me into realization. When it comes to minimalism, one, in particular, strikes me each time.

"For it is easier for a camel to go through the eye of a needle than for a rich man to enter the kingdom of God." Luke 18:22-25

There are two dimensions to being a minimalist. The first, as we have seen in the last few chapters, is that the lack of material things results in clarity. Indeed, that is an important part of the entire prospect of less is best. Clarity leads to many wonderful things. Creativity, freedom, peace, and truth to name just a few. We have seen how this clarity can inspire the movement forward and how it allows the person to go on to bigger and better accomplishments.

The other side of this state of being is the actual process of letting go. Letting go has a tremendous impact on the psyche of a person. In the act of possession, there is a visceral hold that goes on. It is the internal fire that causes the visible smoke of greed. This visceral lock, that latches on to all things we come upon, needs to be released in order for the soul to scale to the next level.

When we release the desire to hold onto things, when we renounce possession beyond what is absolutely necessary, that lock releases and with it the burden that keep us enslaved. The emancipation of the soul is accomplished by the act of coming to terms with the concept of less.

So now you have seen two consequences of less. One is the emancipation of the soul and the other is clarity of the mind. When you live a life that is driven by a soul that is free and a mind that is clear, you become almost superhuman. And this superhuman feeling is one that grows every day as you chose it to do so.

What most people mistakenly assume is that minimalism is about giving away random things. But in actual fact, minimalism is about clearing your cup of the mud that fills it so that you can fill the cup with whatever else you may need.

You must understand that you cannot hold the loaf if you keep your hands busy with the crumbs. And that is essentially the point of being a minimalist. But you won't see that, and you can't see that if you have the wrong priorities filling your eyes. Which is why, conversion to a minimalist's disposition is iterative and repetitive, and happens in stages.

This is your next lesson, then: Do not expect to become a minimalist overnight. You set yourself on a path to it and allow it to move you along the path until you get to a point that you start to feel its effects and its benefits.

One of the things that was unlocked when I became a minimalist was that there was a change in the flavor of my ego. With most of us, our definition of who we are is essentially our ego. If you want to understand this life and move on to greater things, one of the aspects of yourself that needs to be jettisoned is your ego. Easier said than done, though.

One of the ways to get a hold of that ego and release it from your self-definition is to be able to experience minimalism because the ego pretty much uses things and objects to define itself. Why do people want to buy a BMW or Ferrari instead of an unknown model? Let's put cost aside. Assume you could easily afford the most expensive one. What is it about the BMW or Ferrari that a person who has not embraced minimalism go after? Well the BMW helps him define who he is, it acknowledges that he has made certain achievements presumably to get there.

When you practice minimalism over time, it helps to erode your ego and that erosion brings truth into focus. Again, minimalism speaks to greater clarity and focusing on the truth is a brand of clarity.

When the ego vanishes, what's left is typically not fooled by the gimmicks out there. No advertisements to make you thinner, or prettier is going to get you to feel bad about yourself. No sports car advertisement is going to make you feel that your life has been droning on, and no failure is going to feel catastrophic.

The annihilation of the ego made me realize that the mistakes I make in the pursuit of an objective were just ways from which to learn how not to do something. Before that, mistakes used to be embarrassing. Having an ego is such a burden, and when you clean house, the ego eventually gets taken out too.

For now, these simple steps and lessons are all you need to get started. A heads-up to let you know what to expect and to get you on your way. But I believe each person is the master of his own path. You, and you alone, need to make the choices that you face in which to better your journey and life. I can't do it for you, nor can anyone else. All I can do; all anyone can do to help you is share experiences in the hopes that you find something relevant to your objective in life. Something that resonates within you. Something that stirs hope and vision for you.

The best thing that I learned about myself was that before I embarked on this simplistic living, I always needed something external to make me feel better internally. I needed a big car, a big house, a better yard than my neighbor's, a nicer bike than my friend, and so on. Although short-lived, there was always something I could buy to make the evening better or the weekend sweeter. But when I became a true minimalist, I no longer felt the need to go to the mall for retail therapy. I had seen the truth. The truth that material objects do not bring true joy and fulfillment.

As a minimalist, the common argument against, or rather the fear among those who oppose it, is the uncertainty of all of it. Somehow most people think that living the life of a minimalist exposes me, and those who rely on me, to uncertainty, and therefore risk. But that is not the case at all. There are things in this universe that work in ways that we are not used to. Universal forces that are hard for many to grasp onto and understand. This universal power is especially difficult to comprehend when we are more concerned with things that do not really matter, than with those that do.

Often times we get what we worry about the most. Your path always arcs towards what your eyes gaze upon. If you look at and focus on all of the things that could go wrong, one of them, or more, will materialize. When you minimize all the things around you, and you gain clarity and faith, things tend to not go wrong unnecessarily.

I now feel good about myself the way I am. And that has made me smile more often, cry less - almost never in fact and then only when I am so happy that the tears are that of joy. It has made me come to appreciate the abundance that life offers me. Beforehand, when I was defined by greed, ego, and materialism I was indeed focusing on the crumbs. Now, the bread is there whenever I need it.

CHAPTER 8
LESS CLUTTER IN THE MIND WITH MEDITATION

"Perfection is achieved, not when there is nothing more to add, but when there is nothing left to take away."
~ Antoine de Saint-Exupery

We are not our minds, bodies, or things. With less clutter in the mind you will be able to focus on simplicity. Here are some tips on meditation and living in the now. Both provide a host of benefits and will make you more productive, happier, and will also raise your vibrations. Read on for some ideas:

Importance of Meditation

For thousands of years, people have been using meditation to quiet their minds and find inner harmony. Meditation helps you concentrate, increases your self-awareness, and helps to fight stress by facilitating the ability to relax and cope with life's problems. Meditation can help insomnia, IBS, PMS, anxiety and panic attacks as well as helping it to control migraines. Studies have shown that meditation can help us in our professional and personal lives.

Meditation Helps You Keep Your Thoughts Under Control

Our minds help us to consciously analyze, plan and communicate ideas. These abilities have helped us to achieve our success and have gotten us to where we are in life today. However, despite the fact that the brain helps us reason, relate to others, and be creative, if we don't learn how to switch it off, it eventually can overwhelm us. If we don't control our thoughts, they can pester us with fear of failure, negative thoughts about our appearance, or worry about opinions that others might have about us. Meditation helps us to quiet this chatter, bringing us relief about these anxieties.

Meditation is for everyone, not just yogis, mystics or philosophers, and here are some tips on how to do it:

Create a Meditation Space

It helps to meditate in the same space every day. Even if you don't have a spare room to meditate in, you can set up a corner or peaceful area in a quiet room that can be reserved for this purpose. You can add a special chair or listen to tranquil sounds like classical music. When you keep the same area for meditation, your brain will learn to associate it with peaceful feelings as soon as you get into the area, putting you into the mindset for meditation.

Learn to Meditate in Other Places

If you simply don't have a quiet area in your home to meditate regularly, there are other places suitable for meditation. If there is nice weather outside, go to the local park. The most important thing to bear in mind is that you want to find a quiet spot where you won't be interrupted. Listen to peaceful music, wear clothes that are comfortable and loose, and stay warm.

Meditate on the Fly

Once you get the hang of meditating, you can really meditate anywhere. (As long as you are not driving or operating heavy machinery, of course.) You can meditate on the subway or train, a bus, or anywhere in between.

Meditation Postures

Seated: You can use a chair, bench or stool to do this posture. Sit up with your back straight, while holding your head and spine in alignment. Rest your hands on your knees or the arms of your chair. Keep your thighs parallel to the floor, and try not to lean against the back of the chair if it has a back.

Cross Legged: Sit on the floor while crossing your legs. Sit upright with your back straight and your head and spine aligned while resting your hands on your knees.

Kneeling Posture: Kneel on the floor with your knees together, buttocks on your heels and your toes almost touching. Keep your back straight, again your head and spine in alignment. Rest your palms on your thighs, and if it feels more comfortable, put a cushion on the backs of your heels.

Lying Down Posture: All you have to do for this posture is lie down on a carpeted floor, towel or mat. Keep your legs straight but relaxed, and let your arms rest comfortably by your sides. This is a great posture if you need to relax or de-stress, but be careful not to fall asleep!

Practice Mindfulness

Mindfulness is a great way to begin meditating. Too many of us run on autopilot, "sleepwalking" our actions through the day, unaware of what is happening around us. Mindfulness helps you to pause your thoughts and reclaim each moment of the day.

To develop mindfulness, you should keep yourself completely in the present moment, notice every sensation and every detail about what is going on around you. Take writing a letter – notice everything about it – the smell of the fresh sheet of paper, the feel of the paper against your hand, the weight of the pen and the feeling of it resting between your fingers. To cultivate mindfulness, try this meditation:

1. Pull your mind away from wherever it is, and purposefully concentrate on whatever you are doing at the moment. Whatever you are doing – walking, eating, taking a shower, begin to do it with all of your senses. Smell the air around you, feel the water against your skin in the shower, taste every mouthful of food you are eating. Ask yourself "what am I doing?" "what am I experiencing and feeling?"
2. After doing this for a little while, chances are your mind will begin to distract you. This is perfectly fine! Notice the thoughts that come up, but don't follow them. With practice, you will be able to let them go and bring yourself gradually back to the present. Keep this good thing going for as long as you can.

Importance of the Now

Most of the time, we are thinking about the past – either fondly or with regret. Or we are longing, or worrying about the future and planning for it. This isn't always a bad thing, having memories is obviously important, and it is good to plan or develop a contingency plan for the worst case scenario.

The problem with living in the past and future is that we live there, and as places and people become regular things, they become repetitive. Research tells us that if we don't claim our thoughts, we are literally only paying one percent of our attention to the here and now.

The real problem arises when our mind roams freely – we subconsciously think that the past is the present. Past experiences, thoughts, and emotions dictate our current behavior. This automation of behavior guided by the past creates our present, our everyday life.

Then there is the future. We are constantly wandering into the future, thinking “what if?” This distracts us, and we lose focus on what is happening now. When we lose focus, doing our tasks now become more of a burden, frustrating us.

As mentioned before, the universe is comprised of energy, and this energy responds to your energy. When your energy is focused on the past, and the “what ifs” you haven't even bothered to show up to the present universe. The universe won't bother to respond to your lack of energy.

Also, when you pay attention to the now, your experience changes. Whether you call it “the zone,” “focus,” “single-mindedness” it’s all the same. We operate at maximum performance when we are concentrating on what we are doing right here, right now. When you are in the flow, things flow for you. You might find that you are in the right place at the right time, and you are in fact the right person.

When you channel more energy into “now” the universe will respond now. If your energy is scattered all over the place, the universe won't have much to return. When you are more present, this gives you presence. It is easier to attract events and people that are more positive.

Seize control of the present. Use meditation to pause your thoughts when your mind is wandering and bring it back to now. Meditation will give you the discipline that is required to do this, and it is easy to start. Simply see a little more, feel a little more, hear a little more, and smell and taste more of where you are at. Do it now, before you even go on to the next paragraph! Take the time. You will be glad you did. Trust me!

CHAPTER 9
WHAT DO CAMPERS, HOTELS AND RESORTS HAVE IN COMMON?

"Simplicity involves unburdening your life, and living more lightly with fewer distractions that interfere with a high quality life, as defined uniquely by each individual."
~ Linda Breen Pierce

Many people love and thoroughly enjoy camping, and staying at hotels and resorts. Why do you think that is? Besides the getting away and adventure aspect of it, I believe that seasonal campsites are often times sold-out, and have waiting lists because people like the simplicity that campers (and hotels and resorts) have to offer. Hotel rooms don't have any clutter in them, whatsoever. They don't have junk piled up in the corners. You don't have to worry about tripping over things. You don't have memorabilia, in hotel rooms, that you seemingly hold onto.

Memorabilia that makes you sad more than brings you joy. I use to hold onto things that were once my grandmother's because I felt that in keeping these things, I would feel closer to her, but in reality, these objects just made me sad every time I looked at them. Check yourself and your emotions in regards to the things you are holding onto. If something brings you true joy and happiness, then keep it, but if you feel neutral, guilty, weighed down, obligated or sad about something, get rid of it.

Holding onto and collecting things, a lot of time comes from fear. Fear of the unknown. Fear that you may one day need it. Fear of an uncertain future. Fear of not having enough. Fear is often the driving force behind not being able to rid yourself of unnecessary stuff. We feel that what we own, our possessions, contributes to our worthiness. The more we have, the more valuable we are. So we think. It's a false perception and it's not true. Storage units are a prime example of this. In years past, storage units did not exist, and now you can find them everywhere and they are filled to capacity. People may a hefty monthly fee to store things that they think they may need, someday.

When people go camping or vacationing at a hotel, or resort, they pack up just what they need and leave the rest behind. This allows them to feel lighter and carefree. Campgrounds are packed with campers from near and far. Many people have campers in campgrounds just a few miles from their home. They leave their large homes that are filled with stuff, every weekend, and stay in their simple camper and live a minimalist lifestyle and they love it. They keep going back to it as often as they can, not even knowing that what they are craving is a simpler lifestyle. What draws a lot of people to camping, or enjoying a stay at a hotel or resort is the carefree feeling these things have to offer. A nice, clean, and organized area that allows for rest and relaxation. Clutter, stuff, and things are distractions and they can hold us back.

I know a couple who previously owned two homes. One

home was used as a camp, like a getaway. It was a small cabin and they retreated there as often as they could. Their cabin was simple and only had the necessities needed. They didn't store their stuff there. They didn't have duplicates of things they didn't need. Their little cabin just had a bed, nightstand, small kitchen, bathroom, and living room with a small bookshelf and laptop. It was cute and cozy. It looked like minimalists lived there and they liked it that way. They intentionally kept it that way because of the way it felt. They could relax there. They found that they were happier there than in any other place they spent their time. Their time at home was okay, but it wasn't as joyful and carefree as the time they spent at their cabin. They often times felt overwhelmed while they were at home. They wanted to figure out what the difference was. After a lot of reflection, they decided to transform their home into a space that felt like a retreat. Why should they have to leave their home to feel more joyful and happy? They asked themselves questions. What were the differences between their home and cabin? What was it about the cabin that they liked? What was it about their home that they felt the need to escape from? They wanted to figure it out. The answers all pointed to simplicity. They decided to take the necessary steps to simplify their lives. They decided to go room by room and get rid of the stuff that they really didn't need. They decided to make their home into their retreat. They sold their cabin and began living the minimalist lifestyle in their own home. And to their surprise, it worked! When they'd get discouraged, they'd remind themselves of their 'why'. All of the reasons why they were moving in this direction. You have to know your whys in order to succeed at accomplishing a goal. They told me that it took about a year to get to where they wanted to be with it. It took discipline to get rid of stuff they had accumulated throughout their entire lives, but in doing so they sensed a freedom and joy like they never had before. They both told me that they are the happiest and healthiest they've ever been.

CHAPTER 10
ALL YOU NEED IN A BAG

"There are two ways to be rich: One is by acquiring much, and the other is by desiring little."
~ Jackie French Koller

Minimalism doesn't mean that you have to fit all of your stuff in one bag, but it definitely gives you something to think about because many minimalists live this way and sing praises about it. Minimalism is, however, about possessing only the essentials. The bare minimum to get by in a way that works for you.

For me, one of the things I got rid of on my journey to minimalism was my smartphone. I had had a smartphone for more than ten years and it had become a part of my life. That was before the ability to get email on it. Then came the Blackberry and a whole new world of push email entered my already busy life. At that time, it was an amazing thing for me to be able to work through lunch.

My family tolerated it but did not like it one bit.

As the models got snazzier and more advanced, I upgraded. Almost every year, because suddenly the latest feature was something that I had to have and without it, life seemed incomplete. For years, I could not have a complete conversation with members of my family without being interrupted by an email, a text message, a chat message or something along those lines. As I think back, it feels absolutely ghastly, and I'm a bit embarrassed at how much I allowed my phone to own and control me. Of course, it was I who was truly in control, but looking back it didn't feel as though that was true. I constantly felt the urge to check it.

When I went through the transformation, I got rid of my smartphone and settled for a simple calls/text message kind of phone. Nothing sexy about it, just functional. I still receive emails, but not on my phone. I get my emails on my laptop that I crank up only during my working hours. Otherwise, my laptop is not even on the table. It's packed away in my bag.

The Bag as the Focal Point

I keep my bag as the focal point of my quest to own as little as possible. Everything I own, and this includes my clothes, and my sleeping gear fits into and onto my eighty-liter backpack. Within that bag, there is also another small backpack that I use when I am out and about. I carry my laptop and camera in there when I am not traveling.

At this point, I have managed to get it down to such a point that if it doesn't fit in the bag, I don't need it. And that works out pretty well. My bed, as I mentioned earlier went from a posturpedic memory mattress to a straw mat that rolls and latches onto my backpack. In the summer I hang that matt out in the sun on a daily basis. When it gets a little worn, I just replace it.

Essentially all of the things I need have to do with personal hygiene, nutrition, rest, and work. When you look at it this way it becomes obvious that if you stick to what you are designed to do, everything else is such a waste. As long as I have shelter and a place to sleep at night and recharge my batteries safely; as long as I have what I need to eat my food and meals, as long as I have what I need to work, I truly do not need anything else. I can carry the pressure cooker and dishes in my bag, and my spouse can carry the induction cooker. But for now, it's stored in the kitchen. When we made the purchase we made sure it fit in our bags. If it didn't fit, it wasn't necessary.

We do travel at times and that's one of the benefits we have been able to enjoy more as minimalists. We have the extra funds and time to do so now. In the past, if we traveled, it was by air exclusively because we needed to get there and rush back. Time was a major consideration. But we have also learned to stop and smell the roses as they say. In doing that we have been able to make friends with people from all walks of life and we have become all the richer for it.

Traveling (and packing) is easier and more affordable when you adopt the minimalist lifestyle. You will also completely lose the fear of losing your stuff. You won't have to worry about keeping your valuables safe from a thief or fire. That worry will be completely gone, never to return. Not having attachments is a freedom in itself, but not having to worry about you things, is a joy that you can't understand until you do it.

CHAPTER 11
USING DISCIPLINE TO SIMPLIFY YOUR LIFE

"You say, 'If I had a little more, I should be very satisfied.' You make a mistake. If you are not content with what you have, you would not be satisfied if it were doubled."
~ Charles Spurgeon

Most dictionaries will tell you in one way or another that discipline is the act of doing something that you don't feel like doing. That definition covers a lot of ground and within its imagery you get the notion that the effort to do what you need to is nonexistent when there is no discipline involved. There is some truth to looking at it that way, but it is incomplete. Because discipline covers thinking as well. You have to apply discipline to what you are thinking. Because thoughts do become actions when left to their own devices. It is discipline that moves fantasy into imagination. If you find that most of your thoughts are self-defeating or bias in nature, then you need to have the discipline to curb those thoughts and change them.

Discipline can be applied to both tangible actions and as well as intangible mental processes. Tangible outcomes refer to things that can be perceived by the five senses, while intangible processes refer to things like thoughts that go through a person's mind. Tangible and intangible form a dance that should be centered around balance but not necessarily constantly centered there. From a simplistic perspective, this definition would suffice. However, for the purposes of analyzing your career and plotting a new trajectory, the discipline that is required is one with a much higher intensity. Thus, it requires a more sensitive definition.

The Three Facets of Discipline

There are three facets to the discipline we seek.

The first is the discipline that aligns our actions to our rational thought. You can think of this as the discipline that gets you to move thought (noumenal) to action which manifests physical results (phenomenal).

The second is a discipline to hold our primal instincts in check. This is where a lot of us get into trouble. The idea of eating too much, for instance, is something that is within us. We need the discipline to move that equilibrium.

The third and final one is the discipline to think, cogitate and pay attention to what is real and what is necessary, versus what is not real, unimportant, or untrue.

These three facets of discipline, as simple as they sound, are some of the hardest things that a human being could possibly undertake to do. But with time and effort, it is very possible to achieve. However, if you are under the impression that this book will outline a series of steps that will magically imbue discipline upon you so that you wake up tomorrow morning with the superhero abilities that are attributed to discipline I'm afraid you're wrong. Discipline, just like anything else, takes practice. Work discipline into a habit and your life will be amazing. Any successful person you know or admire has learned this skill one way or another, and you can too.

Any behavioral change required to be installed in the human psyche requires two aspects to be accomplished, one is phenomenal the other is noumenal, as we have seen in other areas when dealing with the human condition. For the purpose of this book, within the context that we speak, phenomenal refers to things that are tangible and noumenal refers to things that are intangible.

Recall in the earlier part of the book, we discussed the energy economics that all of us have running in the background. For the most part, these energy economic methods are fairly spot on and serve us well. Imagine if you require 300 calories to walk from point A to point B. You are currently in Point A and your lunch is located at point B. You know that your lunch will only serve you 200 calories. If your body is fine-tuned, it's going to know right then and there, that that particular trip is not worth it.

That's the basics. Now add on top of that the typical inflation of the effort and diminishing return equation. The mind is left to calculate the possible effort and energy to execute the trip, and it is tasked with figuring out what the chances are that the energy source will be there when you arrive. If the mind feels that there is only a 50% chance, that equation is going to get skewed even more.

Now, this has been a rather long, yet simplistic illustration, but that is essentially how the mind works. We get lazy to do something because we inflate the effort required or diminish the return and compute that the effort is not worth it, so we sit on our laurels waiting for the next opportunity to come along.

Behavioral Change Using Discipline

To change this, what psychologists call behavioral change, is actually doing one of three things. You can either completely disregard the conclusion drawn by your subconscious, or your inaction, or laziness in this instance, and apply the effort to do it - this is blind discipline loyal only to acting on an objective; or you can change your thinking about the probability of the return; or you could think and reflect about the actual effort required and possibly automate, mechanize, or somehow reduce the necessary input - this requires mental energy expended.

So again, you simply need to change your thinking about the probability of the return. Often times if we can't see instant results, we tend to put off taking action, by simply being deliberate in how we think about it, we can change the outcome. Good things take time. Transformation takes time. Success takes time. In either case, the various faculties of the mind need to be realigned so that the new equilibrium can be achieved. It is discipline, as we have seen, that moves this equilibrium.

Anything worth having requires discipline. In order for goals to be reached and fulfilled people have to incorporate discipline into their lives. There is no way around it. It may be uncomfortable and you may not like it at first, but if you want to see results you have to be strong. You have to strengthen your willpower.

With success comes discipline and you will have to be disciplined in order to form a new way of thinking, which will lead to a new and improved lifestyle. As with all bad habits that we eventually break, your freedom from it lies just around the corner. Don't give up! Keep moving towards your goal because you will reach it! So exciting!

CHAPTER 12
MINIMALISM SUCCESS

"Simplicity is the ultimate sophistication."
~ Leonardo daVinci

If you have no discipline, minimalism success will elude you and it will seem like you aren't getting anywhere or reaching your goals. Discipline is what gets you to do the things that are necessary in the pursuit of success. If you do what is necessary, then success is just a matter of time. The good thing is that all of us has utilized discipline in one way or another to get the results we wanted; to reach a desired goal. You may have used discipline without being fully aware that that was what you were doing, but nonetheless, you were using it. Once you realize this and become deliberate with the benefits of discipline, your life can be absolutely incredible. Discipline is a tool, and you are capable of using it on a regular basis to fulfill and reach your dream of simplifying.

In many situations, people slip over and over again and fail in their attempts to be successful or build a life based on their goals. They make the mistakes, they seemed to have learned from their mistakes, time and time again, but they still can't seem to make it work because they don't have the discipline to execute what they have learned. To many people, success and ultimate goal reaching is still a mystery.

Being a winner, and successful at reaching your goals is not so much about hard work as it is about having the right mindset and pursuing a course of action that is consistent with the manifestation of the desired outcome. This requires discipline.

The psychology involved in putting one's self on the winning trajectory begins with the clarity of the desired outcome followed by the discipline to refrain from paying any attention to distractions that may arise along the way. Distractions are ever present, whether one chooses to be a successful, or one is indifferent, distractions are a part of life and they always will be. The sooner you learn to overcome the many distractions that life is constantly throwing at you the better off you will be.

There are eight elements where you must apply discipline to in order to jumpstart your minimalism success:

Mindset

Mindsets are everything and if you want to understand the psychology behind the being successful at simplifying your life, you are first going to have to get comfortable with various categories of mindsets and the means to mold them to your conscious desires. Molding mindsets are done with consistent work and unrelenting discipline.

The typical mindset required to be successful is one that is constantly self-reflecting, and doing what is necessary at every stage. It is also not doing things that are unnecessary because time is a precious commodity when success is the goal. The key to mindsets is that they have to be neutral or positive - never negative.

Perception

You will also need to evaluate your current habits of perception, especially perception of yourself. Most unsuccessful people have a poor perception of everything around them. They can also keep themselves so busy with unnecessary things that they never reach their goals. In order to be successful you need to have faith that everything can go your way, and in the meantime, you need to see things for what they really are and then take action to make the necessary course corrections.

Now, this is a slightly complex concept because there are two versions of perception that you need to contend with. There are two because they are two sides of the same coin. The first side is the perception you have of yourself and how that contends with how you want to see yourself in the future. What type of person do you want to be? How do you want to live? The second is how you feel others perceive you. That second one is a little complicated. It is not what others perceive of you - certainly not - because you can't possibly know what they see you as. Instead, it is what you think they see you as that has to balance the other side of the coin. Perception is a big part of satisfying your goals.

Reflection

The next foundation that you need, is the concept of reflection. If you didn't already know it, reflection is one of the key elements that every single highly successful person uses. They don't just do it weekly or sporadically. The true greats either do it daily or they are in a constant state of reflection. Reflection helps you to look at things the way they are and not the way you think they are. Reflection helps you to transcend notions and bias and if you do it correctly it helps you to see things that you ordinarily would miss.

So many times we think we know what others are thinking or why they are doing what they are doing. We make assumptions that just aren't true. We also think things about ourselves that just aren't true. It is finding the truth that will set you free. For spiritual people, the Bible or some other book may hold the truth for you. The truth is we are all powerful, capable, and lovable beings. We are all one even though at times we perceive to be separate. We are capable of living the life we intend for ourselves.

Happiness

The next foundation is often missed but is a highly critical pillar, nonetheless, and that is the desire and willingness to be happy. Have you ever seen a sore winner? Or a sad winner? No. If you think that the winners are happy just because they won, you are wrong. The opposite is true. They won and will continue to be winners because they are happy. This applies a bit to the Law of Attraction and I wrote a lot about that in my book "Get It Up: 101 Ways to Raise Your Vibration, Reduce Stress, Depression, & Anxiety, Increase Joy, Peace, & Happiness and Attract Abundance Automatically!"

Being happy is also a mindset and altering your mindset to include happiness, or completely creating a new mindset that prioritizes happiness, is not an arduous task. Mindsets can be changed easily if you practice discipline.

Strong Mind

A strong mind is a prerequisite to building and keeping the right set of mindset towards minimalism. Not all of us are born with the propensity toward a strong mind. But that's not a prerequisite. It's a bonus. If you have a weak mind, and you will know it if you do, then your first task, before you do anything else would be to take steps to fortify your mind. A robust mind, able to withstand distractions, able to synthesize purpose, and willing to undergo pain, is what we all aspire to build for ourselves. You can practice having a strong mind through meditation or some other form of mental focus. Once your mind learns to obey you, you will be on your way to success, but this takes practice. Transformation takes time.

Being a winner can be about hard work if you like, or it can be about disciplined work. Winners are people who seem to handle gargantuan tasks with grace and ease. You don't see them sweating and groaning. These are the people who overcome the highest obstacle with the lowest struggle; magnify the simplest visions to gain the best outcomes, and do it all with grace and poise. And you can accomplish this with discipline. Successful people start somewhere with their goal in mind, then take action, and you can too!

Habits

Forty to fifty percent of all that we do and accomplish happens because of this thing called habit. How and when we brush our teeth; the way we comb our hair; the drive to work; our initial response to unexpected stimuli, and much, much more are driven by processes beyond our conscious observation. For simplicity, we refer to the area beyond conscious observation as the subconscious.

Things like habits reside in the subconscious space of the mind while willful acts reside in the conscious space of mind. This willful discipline that's in the conscious state of mind has a counterpart that resides within the subconscious state of mind and that is disciplined habit - or an act where we used discipline to kick off what has now become a habit.

The great thing about habits is that they remove all perception of effort from the conscious mind and transfers the tasks to accomplish something to the subconscious mind. This frees up the conscious mind to do something else. Habits are key and discipline and minimalism can become one of them. When you learn to create your own habits instead of letting nature and the circumstances around you form them for you, you will own your power and discover that you are indeed the captain of your own ship.

Character

Character is a combination of conscious elements and subconscious elements. We define character as the moral qualities of a person's thoughts, words, and deeds. Each person's character is unique, and they are unique because they are driven by different levels of stimuli when their character is tested. To illustrate, let's say the mark of character is a person not stealing money - regardless of how large or small the amount. The amount shouldn't make a difference.

An exercise you can do to reflect on character is to write out who you want to be. What characteristics do you wish to instill? Writing them out can help you become aware of who you want to become. Organized, clean, honest, sincere, faithful, giving, kind, responsible, trustworthy, reliable, etc. Once you know in detail who you want to become you can start acting deliberately. If you want to start simplifying your life, then you need to start getting rid of things that no longer serve you.

Those are the eight characteristics that you can mold with discipline to help you succeed. Doing so will help elevate your game to the next level, not only in simplifying your life, but in all other areas as well.

CHAPTER 13
LESS IS BEST TESTIMONIES

"I don't think it matters what brought you to your minimalist lifestyle. What matters is the freedom that is found from it."
~ Unknown

Please find below testimonies from people who have simplified their lives. Reading other people's stories can help us relate, as well as give us helpful tips and ideas. Knowing that others have done it, can inspire us to do the same.

Testimony 1

I was a young child when my parents got divorced. Four years old to be exact. I didn't want my dad to leave and I didn't understand why he was packing his stuff up in his dark blue, Chevy, El Camino. I cried harder with each trip he made out to the truck and I pleaded with him not to go, but to my dismay, he said he had to. I ran to my parent's bedroom window and watched him, through tears, drive out of the driveway and down the road. My one-year-old brother, lay in a crib just a few feet away. We only saw my dad occasionally after that. Once every other month or so. My dad's girlfriend got pregnant right away, so they got married and started a family of their own. My brother and I were raised by my hardworking, single mother until I graduated from high school. She was heartbroken for a very long time and hardened her heart to men. She did everything a dad would have done. Worked two jobs, mowed the law, tended the garden, shoveled the driveway. Back then, fathers were not forced to pay child support and my dad couldn't afford to pay with his new wife and three kids, so we struggled financially, year after year. My brother and I didn't have toys. I had a rock collection though, that I thoroughly enjoyed, and a porcelain music box that I treasured. More recently I saw the same exact music box at a large flea market we have in our area. To walk into this flea market is to go back in time. Even with all of the miscellaneous items that jam packed this flea market, this music box caught my attention and held it. I couldn't take my eyes off from it. I remembered. I picked up the music box and slowly twisted the circular underbelly of it. It played "Raindrops Keep Falling on My Head". The entire flea market and all of the people shopping around me disappeared. It was just me and my old music box and I felt sad. I feel sad right now writing about it. I think my childhood was a bit sad. Oh, my mother, and brother loved me very much and the three of us had a wonderful relationship, still do, but I don't think I quite understood why, or how my dad could leave us. Although my dad and I have a good relationship now, and I don't blame him at all,

I think there was a piece of me that was broken. My husband walked up behind me as I stood in front of the spinning music box and I told him I had one as a child. He enthusiastically asked if I wanted to get it. I thought about it as I stared at this very familiar piece of my childhood and said "no". I didn't have much growing up, so as an adult, and with kids of my own, I struggled with throwing anything away. And I mean anything. My children had so many toys and even the cheapest, smallest toys, you know the free ones that come with the Happy Meals? Even those, I couldn't throw away. It was out of control. Until one day my husband and I decided that we wanted to move closer to our parents, therefore, we put our house on the market. Our house sold in three weeks so we had a lot of packing to do in a short amount of time. Our house was a ranch style home and we truly believed that we would be able to get it all in one large U-Haul. We rented the largest U-Haul that they rent out and got busy. We left dozens of trash bags out for the trash truck each week and we made truckload trips to the Goodwill with furniture, clothes, toys, etc. With everything we got rid of, we would definitely be able to fit everything in the large U-Haul truck. We had no doubt. Well, you guessed it, when the time came it took us two trips with the U-Haul truck and we still had stuff we were packing in our friend's and family's trucks and cars. It was absolutely silly; the time and energy we put into moving all of this stuff that we thought we needed. It's funny how we justify the definition of "need" when we are looking at something that we can't seem to let go of. It took me a long time to learn that our stuff doesn't define us, and that it actually holds us back. I read somewhere (I think in a Feng Shui book) that even if you have a storage unit half way across the world, the stuff in that storage unit affects you and weighs you down. Holds you back. Even though you can't see it, it's there and it affects your creativity and freedom. Like I said, it took a long time for me to get to where I wanted to be with stuff. It was a slow process. But I got there slowly but surely. I keep reading blogs, articles, and books on minimalism and it kept feeling right for me. So I just started getting rid of stuff. Little by little and item by item. My life has been so much freer ever since. I have more time now than I ever had before and more freedom to do what I want to do. It's been great and I recommend that everyone, to at least, give it a try. ~ Sally

Testimony 2

I felt a slow transformation and renewing of my mind after I started attending church regularly. Part of this transformation was the desire to simplify my life. I felt it deep within my bones. I'm not going to lie though; it was extremely challenging and a lot harder than I thought it would be. I knew that I wanted to simplify, and I knew that minimalism was calling me, but it took me years to truly get into the groove with it. I started by getting rid of things I knew that I didn't want. I made several trips to donation drop-off locations. About once a month I was donating full trunk loads of stuff. It wasn't easy at first. And it didn't get any easier, at first, either. I held onto everything and let memories flood back as to how I got it, from when and where, to how I felt about the person and the day it was given to me. Each object held dozens of memories, thoughts, and feelings. So, as you can imagine, it was taking a lot of time and energy. I also had a hard time getting rid of books. I'd pick up each book and flip through it. Some I'd start to read even. It was no productive at all. It took me about three full weeks to go through my books, and mostly because I had to flip through each one. I got rid of 116 books during that time, but had a lot more to go. Why we feel that we need to hold onto things is beyond me. We can't take things with us and this is where I was coming from in wanting to simplify my life. I had heard of people putting all they own in one suitcase and I was inspired by this. I knew that a sense of freedom was to be found beyond this goal of mine. But I couldn't figure out why it was so hard. Two years of getting rid of stuff, and I still had way more stuff to discard. What I still owned would fill a dump truck and none of the stuff had much value to it. It was just stuff that I couldn't bear to part with. As I continued to study minimalism, I kept feeling called to it. So I decided to get serious. I went room by room each and every Saturday. It would take most of the day, too. I'd go through each room one at a time, and clean out what I didn't think I needed. Each Saturday, I felt as though I did pretty good, but come the next Saturday I'd do it all over again and get rid of even more stuff. I found that I wasn't missing anything that I had gotten rid of either. It got easier and easier. Each Saturday I'd clean out more as if I was just starting fresh. I gave myself a number for each item, for example, I allowed myself only five bracelets, five pairs of earrings, and five necklaces. Once I had the number that I had decided on, I'd lay them all out and then decide what to keep. Eventually I got down to owning only four pairs of shoes, five pairs of pants, ten shirts, five sweaters, and a few dresses. I only kept things that felt absolutely wonderful to wear. Anything that I didn't wear or that was questionable, I got rid of. I canceled all of my magazine subscriptions. I allowed myself to own 20 books but still feel the need to own fewer and use the resources of the library instead. I also want to utilize my kindle for the books that I always want to have access to at my fingertips. I think minimalism can be different for each person and that you have to keep going until you feel satisfied. Minimalism is about not needing to be attached to stuff and to have faith that all of your needs will always be met. It's also about the environment and not being wasteful. It's about riding yourself of things that are taking up too much of your time. Life is short, and you want to enjoy life's experiences and not be a slave to materialism and things. Life has been wonderful since I've joined my church and continued to learn more of The Bible. I can't believe I waited this long for the life-giving rewards that come from it. Not only have I cleaned out my home, but I've also cleaned out my mind, my heart, and my soul. It's been amazing. I have more money than I've ever had before, I've had more peace than I've ever had before, I've had more courage than I've ever had before, and so it goes in all other areas of my life as well. Minimalism has been a huge part of the freedom my soul rejoices in every day. ~ Alicia

Testimony 3

My minimalism testimony happened after my family and I suffered from a house fire. We were sort of forced into the minimalist lifestyle and surprisingly it has stuck. Having our home destroyed by fire, was life changing, to say the least. It put everything into perspective. We were lucky to be alive and to have it happen as it did so that everyone, including our pets, got out in time. Someone was looking out for us. My wife, three children, dog, and 2 cats were fine. The fire was caused by a faulty outlet, although we didn't know it at the time, and thankfully it didn't happen while everyone was sleeping. I feel so blessed because of the way it happened and that our lives were spared. After the firemen finished putting the fire out, we were told that everything was destroyed. Nothing was salvageable. Everything that we had ever owned was completely gone. We stood in shock and awe. What were we going to do? A lot of stuff ran through our mind. We kept calling out things that were in there that we wished we could've saved. My dad's trophies, our children's baby pictures, the blanket that my grandmother made, the letters my wife and I sent to each other when we were dating. These attachments now caused us pain. We were sad and depressed for months it seemed. We left the fire scene with nothing but the clothes on our backs... and each other. Thankfully. Although I felt depressed, I couldn't help but feel so grateful and blessed and thankful. My heart exploded with gratitude that my family was okay, and the fact that it could've been a lot worse. We had each other. We slowly picked the pieces up and our church gave us money to get new clothes. I felt so thankful that we had our church family. They were so supportive. We learned so much from this devastating and scary experience and I was determined to not let it happen again. While I was waiting at the insurance company, I came across an article in a magazine. The article was on the subject of simplifying. One guy could fit everything he owned in the trunk of his car. Another could fit all of his belongings in two backpacks. I couldn't help but think that if my family had done that we wouldn't have been so devastated. Yes, it would still have been a huge loss and a big adjustment, but I think if we had only lost a backpack of belongings it definitely wouldn't have affected us so negatively. As we moved and started to accumulate the necessities, we thought about it differently than we ever had before. We only purchased what we felt we needed. I think that, yes, we could fit all of our stuff in a pickup truck. Yes, we were forced into this lifestyle, but now that we've done it, we don't want to go back. It's been great. It takes my wife less time to clean the house, it takes us less time to do laundry. We've found more time for each other without all of the distractions that all of old "stuff" took away from us. Don't ask me how or why stuff interferes with your time, but trust me it does. I would have to say that my life now is so much happier than it was before. I guess you could say the fire that burned down our house was a blessing. ~ Toby

Testimony 4

Thank you, Sage, for allowing me to submit my story of how I simplified my life of many things and people that did not benefit me or my soul. This story probably isn't for young people, so if you're a young person you should skip this section. I regret it and chalk it up to a lesson learned, though. I didn't have proper guidance. I didn't know the truth. I was blinded. I didn't listen to my inner being. I didn't listen to my intuition. I didn't listen. When I was a teenager, I babysat, part-time, for a couple who lived not far from me. Tricia and Tony. They had two young children and I liked the convenience of them living so close. I babysat for them for four years and grew close to their entire family. After I graduated from high-school, I decided to take courses at a community college, in my home state, in hopes of saving money. After doing the math, I made the decision to commute during my first two years while taking the core classes I needed to transfer to University. This worked out well because I could continue to work and babysit part time. The couple I babysat for were only 7 and 9 years older than me and I felt as though they were easy to get along with. They were a great looking couple and very active. Half the time I babysat so that they could work-out together, go hiking, biking, etc. and the other half of the time they'd go out partying and dancing. Eventually the time came for me to let them know that I would be leaving within the next couple of months. This didn't come to a surprise to them, as they knew what my plans were all along. One night after they got home from a night out of drinking and dancing, Tony came into the kitchen and jokingly spanked me on the behind, grabbing my butt before pulling his hand away. He said "Now that you're an adult, and will no longer be employed by us, I figured I'd give you a little good luck spanking." Tricia laughed and a look came over her face like she had just had the most brilliant idea. I was horrified and didn't like it one bit. A few nights later, Tricia asked me to stop by. Tony's 30th birthday was coming up and she wanted to give him a birthday present like no other. She wanted to surprise him by fulfilling one of his fantasies. She said they really liked and trusted me, and she asked if I'd consider joining them in the bedroom just one time, for his birthday. I was shocked, and told her that I'd have to think about it. I remember trying to get out of there as quick as possible. I was not going to be a part of this! No way! It felt wrong just thinking about it. Tricia told me to let her know within the week. She kept saying "please" and assured me that it'd be fun, and that because we were all close and trusted each other that everything would be fine. She told me that she knew I thought her husband was attractive because of the way my voice got higher whenever he was around. Did it? I wasn't sure. I went home and wanted to talk to my mother about it, but she was never home, and my father hadn't been around since I was 2 years old, so talking to him wasn't an option. I laid on my bed thinking about what Tricia had asked. Tony was good looking. Once in a while he would walk around without his shirt on and I just about died because he was in such good shape. I should be honored that she asked me right? I had only been with one other boy, but I wasn't a virgin so that wouldn't be a problem. No, no, no. This idea was crazy. Nothing seemed right about it. I told Tricia that I wasn't sure. She told me not to worry about it and that she understood. But she said that she had decided to have a few friends over for dinner to celebrate Tony's birthday and that she was going to send the kids to her mother's house for the night. She hoped that I would just pop in for a little bit, and she asked if I wouldn't mind bringing the salad. I agreed. Phew, I was off the hook. Yes, there would be others there and Tricia must have come to her senses. I was so relieved. When the night came, I put the salad together and went over. There were only a few people there, but I knew everyone. Tricia told me to have a sit and gave me some of her special punch which was a mix of different alcoholic beverages. It was delicious and went down very easily. Everyone was drinking and having a good time and dinner was delicious. The more punch we had, the more we all laughed and giggled. After dinner we all moved into the living room to play a game. As Tony walked past me to the couch he squeezed my behind again, and winked at me. I smiled at him, clearly feeling the effects of the alcohol now. It was messing with my brain because this time I liked it. Tony leaned in and whispered, "maybe you can give me a real birthday present later. Tricia said she wouldn't mind." I found myself replying "Maybe". Maybe? I don't think so. This was not okay and I was not morally okay with it either. I decided I was not going to drink much more because obviously it was getting to me, and obviously I wasn't thinking straight. As the night went on, I could feel Tony looking at me. It was hard not to drink more, because we were playing drinking games. Finally, as everyone was leaving, I got up to leave too. I was tipsy and the room was spinning a bit. I thought my best bet would be to walk home. As I reached for my jacket, Tony put his hand on it and told me to wait just a few minutes as they said goodbye to everyone. Oh my goodness, Tricia must have talked to him. She must have already put this idea in his head. As the last guests left, I reached for my jacket again, and thanked Tricia and Tony for a fun night. "The night doesn't have to be over", Tony said leaning in, "I'm hoping for a little birthday kiss." Tricia looked on in approval. "He only has a 30th birthday once, you know?" The room was continuing to spin as Tony's lips reached mine. His tongue found its way into mine and before I knew what was happening, his hands were all over me. As my hands ran up the inside of his shirt, I had confirmation that his chest was as hard as it looked. Tony took my hand and put it down his pants. Shortly after he lead Tricia and I to their bedroom. "Best birthday ever." He said when we were done as he gently kissed me on the lips. Breakfast was a bit awkward, although we all tried to make it seem like it was just another normal morning like the ones where I'd spend the night because they had gotten home so late. I went home and wondered what and how this had even happened. They say once you cross a line, it's hard to go back. Well I went back to Tricia and Tony's bed on several more occasions. It started to become a regular thing. And I started realizing that all I could think about was Tony. Day and night, he was all that was on my mind. One morning he called and asked if I could come over that night. When I got there, I was surprised to see him waiting at the door with a bouquet of flowers. I was even more surprised to find out that Tricia had taken the kids out-of-state for a family wedding. Tony couldn't go because he had to work the next day. This was the first time we were alone, and it was absolutely incredible. I realized, then and there, that I had fallen absolutely and madly in love. I hope this isn't getting too long, Sage. I know you said it could be as long or as short as I wanted it to be and maybe releasing this is healing in some way. Tony and I continued to meet alone. I told Tricia that I didn't want to participate in the threesomes anymore. Little did she know that it was because I no longer wanted to share him with her. The thought of it now made me nauseous. I knew what we were doing was wrong and I didn't like how it made me feel inside. This was a family that I loved. How could I even consider doing this? But I couldn't help how I felt inside.

You can't help who you love, right? (Only now do I know how wrong that statement is.) Long story short, one wrong deed led to another, and heartache and pain were the only possible outcomes. My mom always said "You can't fly with the eagles if you are hanging out with the turkeys," and "Every decision has a consequence." And I didn't listen. I became pregnant. Tricia and Tony got divorced. People hated us. Tony and I tried to make a go of our new relationship with our newborn son. His party friends now came over to our place. And even partying didn't feel right to me. Once reality set in, it didn't work. It was awful, dysfunctional, untrustworthy, you name it, it wasn't good. I felt guilty when I saw Tricia and the kids. I remembered how good their relationship was before his birthday party. My inner being was dying. Why didn't I listen to my intuition in the first place? If I had just been firm and strong that day, I wouldn't be in the situation I was in. I had had other men who were interested in me back then. Unmarried men! How different my life would be if I would've just stayed strong and listened to the doubt and uncomfortable feeling I had about the whole thing. I never, in a million years, would have imagined myself in a situation such as this. I finally recognized that I was sick from the inside out, and that I literally couldn't take anymore. I couldn't eat. I had no appetite. I lost so much weight that my family was worried about me. I had to take action, for myself and for my son. I knew deep down in my soul that this wasn't going to work. I knew I didn't want to party all the time. I knew that I wanted to go back to school and start getting back on the right path. A path that I knew was there for me. I just had to take action. In my desperation, I cried out to God. I begged him to help me. I didn't know what else to do. Two weeks later, a woman I worked with asked if I wanted to go to church with her. I accepted her offer, and my life hasn't been the same since.

I have learned so much from the Bible and from my church family. Wow, I wished someone had introduced me to this before. It is my goal to raise my child with the knowledge and tools that are available at our fingertips. Others have been through similar challenges and sins, and have repented, learned from them, and come out the other side better because of it. I've since apologized to Tricia and asked for her forgiveness. She knows that we were all responsible in some way. Obviously, she had never meant for it to go as far as it did. I don't think any of us did. The Bible tells us not to sin because sin is not good for us. There is nothing good that can come from it. So in summary, I decided to rid myself of people and things that were not good for my soul. It was a process, but I did it. Eventually I also learned that people and things are not where our satisfaction comes from. Satisfaction and joy can only come from our creator. Two years after regularly going to church, and Bible studies, I paid off my debt and purchased a tiny-home for my son and I. I feel like freer than I ever have. It's true that the truth shall set you free. ~ Tracy

Testimony 5

I simplified my life by getting off social media. That was the start of my minimalist journey. I decided to not use my cell-phone or go on social media for 60 days! My original plan was to see if I could go one day without it, but it ended up lasting 60 days. The first day was the hardest! What a habit it had become, looking at my cell-phone almost every minute of the day it seemed! Wow, I did not realize how much I was really using it. Once I got through the first few days, I felt more and more confident that I could get through another. I felt stronger and stronger with each new day and I even felt like I was getting myself back. It was almost like I had forgotten who I was kind of. I was so attached to that thing. It was freeing. Not seeing the drama that is usually all over the social media sites. I found that I was enjoying my dinners with my family and enjoying the conversation as well. I wasn't getting distracted by social media. I was actually giving people my full attention which felt great, but the downside was that I was now noticing more when others weren't doing the same. I was fully present during conversations with others, but they were not. They were still checking their phones and that was frustrating at times. Also, I lost the need to feel as though I had to check it every second. I told my boyfriend that he wouldn't be able to contact me that way, so he knew not to even try. Before, I always felt like I was going to miss something if I didn't have my phone. If I left the house without it, I would go into a panic mode almost. But once I started not using it, all of these unhealthy feelings disappeared. It was freeing! But it took discipline. Once I accomplished it though, I knew I could use discipline to simplify other areas of my life as well. I started cleaning out stuff that I had originally thought I needed. For example, I had five Michael Kors purses. That's where I started. I gave away three of them right away. When I did this, I knew something was changing inside me because before this I wouldn't have even imagined giving away my MK purses! This led to such a freeing experience. After giving away my treasured and expensive purses, that I had worked hard for, I kept going with all of my other possessions. My clothes, shoes, furniture, jewelry, books. Things now are so much better for me. It's easier to save money, and it's easier to clean and tidy up. Everything just seems easier. Simplifying rocks! ~ Ashley

Testimony 6

How we simplified our lives and are happier because of it. We have three teenage children and live in an old farmhouse. The rooms are oddly shaped and some are very small. Our downstairs consisted of a full bathroom, one bedroom, a laundry room, kitchen, small den, and dining room, and our upstairs consisted of three bedrooms and a full bathroom. For years, we knew that we wanted to simplify our lives and start living smaller. The economy helped us make this decision as well with rising gas and grocery prices. We were tired of living paycheck to paycheck. We decided that we would rent out the upstairs of our home to a family member. We would convert our upstairs to an in-law apartment, and we didn't have to do too much to make it happen. Mostly we had to change our way of thinking! We put a sink, small refrigerator, and set of cupboards on one wall of one of the upstairs bedrooms. This would now be a kitchen, and we put shelves in the closet of that bedroom to convert it to a little pantry. So one bedroom is just that, a bedroom, one bedroom is being used as a living room, and the final bedroom is being used as a kitchen with a refrigerator, sink, microwave, hotplate, and toaster over. We also put a door at the bottom of the stairs just to add to the privacy, but we really didn't need to. We didn't know how it was going to work, at first, because this was a huge change and we lost a lot of living space. In regards to the downstairs, the den became a bedroom, the living room became a bedroom, and we now use the dining room as a small living room with just a loveseat and T.V. It has been an adjustment and we had to get rid of a lot of things, but it has almost been a year now, and we have loved all of the positive rewards that have come from this change. Not only does it take us less time to clean, we are now closer as a family. We are around each other more, so we can communicate more, and be aware of how things are going for each of our children. Even our pets are closer, as funny as that sounds. We rarely saw our cat before, because she'd always be hiding in an upstairs bedroom. Now she is friendly and a lot more social. In reality, you only need to use your bedrooms to sleep, and I found that a couple of our teenagers were using their bedrooms to hideout, or play video games, or be on their computers. Now, although they still do that, we are in close proximity to contribute and be a part of their lives without appearing to be pushy or overbearing. In just walking through our house, we are more present and more available to them. We have more conversations with them. It has been great. When we do laundry, we don't have to make the trip upstairs to put clothes away. We are finding a lot more time and energy for not only our family but for ourselves as individuals. It has created freedom. We have more time to read, relax, take naps, etc. It has been one of the best decisions that we've ever made and in the process, we are continuing to get rid of things that we do not need. Minimalism is our ultimate goal. ~ Steve and Shirley

Testimony 7

Since I decided to become a minimalist, my life has been incredible. Every day (and night for that matter), okay several times a day, I find myself thinking 'I am so happy. Life is incredible! How did I get so lucky?' I feel like it is a freedom of sorts. I don't know how else to explain it. Life is just so good. I use to dream about being a minimalist and it took me longer than I wanted it to because it was hard for me to let go of a lot of my things, but little by little, it got easier because that was the goal. When I first started to get organized, I could not believe how much stuff I had actually collected. For example, I found 36 chap-sticks. Seriously. I found chap-stick on my desk, in the junk draw, in my nightstand, in the kitchen, in a decorative basket in my entryway, in my living room, on my bookshelf, etc. I also put all of my perfumes and body sprays in one place. Before I kept these items in my medicine cabinet, on my bureau, in a hall closet, in my vanity. I had perfumes and body sprays in several locations, so I got organized and ended up counting 27! 27 perfumes and body sprays? It was like every time I went into a department store, I had to stop and test the perfume samples, and then waste a lot of valuable time on trying to decide which one to buy. I gathered 16 things of floss, 62 mini hand-sanitizers from Bath & Body Works, 77 nail polishes, 49 hair elastics, 34 costume jewelry bracelets, 4 pairs of sneakers. The list goes on and on. These are just simple examples of ways that I have wasted my time and money without even realizing it. Just because I was living a bit disorganized. And I consider myself a very neat, clean, and tidy person. I never would've guessed how unorganized I really was. And I found this with pots and pans, dishes, plastic containers, etc. I had 2 griddles, one didn't work great, but it was still stored in the cupboard. Now everything has a place. I learned to get rid of things that I didn't need. I had to think about things differently. I had to repeatedly ask myself what I needed, and when getting rid of stuff that I didn't use or was unsure of, I'd ask myself what was the worst thing that would happen if I didn't have it. Not only do I feel better and happier, I have also had other benefits come out of it that I wasn't expecting. I've started my own business, saved more money than I ever have before, and have signed up for some clubs where I have been some wonderful people and I get to socialize and have fun. Something I wouldn't have had time for before. For some odd reason. I don't know exactly why minimalism works, but it does. My life has never been more rewarding. If you're thinking about minimalism, give it a try. What have you got to lose? Take it from me, life is so good when you simplify. ~ Stacey

Testimony 8

Before I became a minimalist, I was addicted to infomercials. I didn't realize how these advertisers work, how they work their magic, and how they are trained to sell you on anything. Companies spend millions of dollars on advertising because it works! They study us. They get us. They know what makes us tick. They pull us in. They convince us to buy their products whether we need them or not. I paid $240 on three plastic fans. The infomercials made them look amazing. I watched for 30 minutes and they were on sale NOW. I was convinced. I picked up the phone and placed the order. When the fans finally arrived in the mail, I was so excited. The only thing special about this fan is that it tilts up and down. It doesn't even oscillate and go back and forth. It just tilts up and down. Looking at the fans now, from a different perspective, I feel scammed almost. I could've easily gotten three fans for $60 and they would've served the exact same purpose and given the exact same results. I didn't know that I had to start thinking differently before I'd be able the truth. I paid $120 for a bra I saw on an infomercial! Again, they kept talking and giving selling points on why I should pick up the phone and make that call. These infomercials almost make you feel stupid if you don't call. When I started leaning on cleaning out my clutter, I started doing a lot of research and reading a lot of books on minimalism and my way of thinking started to change. I started to see the truth. In my research I found out that so many people have this problem and fall into the infomercial trap. It's human nature and you have to stop yourself and be aware of what is happening. I still, from time to time, almost get sucked in. I think I need something. It seems silly now because I know how it works, but even with knowing and being aware of the selling tactics they use, to make us want something, there have been a couple times where I have almost given in to the pressure. You really have to be strong and disciplined to not let those things suck you in.

Now I try to teach my children what is going on when a commercial comes on in which they make a simple plastic product look absolutely amazing. It's their jobs as advertisers to make us want it, and that is exactly what they do. A lot of people are not fond of car salesmen, because of how they operate, but this is exactly what advertisers are doing to us. I think the more we simplify our lives the easier it becomes. I am happy to say that I no longer pick up the phone and buy things that I don't need. And when I feel tempted, I just say 'Job well done' to the advertising company for doing their job well. Again, many companies spend millions of dollars on advertising because it works and they get the returns they need from them. As for me, I now have three plastic fans that I paid $240 for and that I can't seem to get rid of because of their odd shape. Lesson learned. If you are thinking about becoming a minimalist, you definitely should. Keep in mind that it is a journey and that you will reach your destination if you keep at it and you will be so glad that you did. I have found that there is an amazing sense of freedom. A freedom like no other, really. It's been an amazing experience and I wouldn't want to go back to my infomercials days for nothing. My purchases always brought about feelings of disappointment, guilt, failure, and discontent. I'm so glad that those days are gone. ~ Natasha

CONCLUSION

"Abundance is a process of letting go;
that which is empty can receive."
Bryant McGill

There are multiple reasons behind stripping everything off and returning to the basics. Living a life of simplicity is not about living poorly, it is about living richly and in focus. When we complicate our lives with material objects and addictions, and then strive and stress to feed those addictions, we find that more often than not we step off the right path and life becomes chaotic, busy, lonely, and unfulfilling. These are not the kinds of mistakes that we want to make. Life is too short. Mistakes we make when we are learning are different from the kinds of mistakes we make when greed sets in amidst the lack of clarity.

Go through each room and decide what you truly need. Continue to do this until you are satisfied. And only keep things that bring you immense joy. Things that make your heart sing. You are so worth the freedom and joy that lies behind minimalism.

There are so many benefits to simplifying our lives. The benefits far outweigh the cons.
Here's a list of just a few of the benefits:

- More time for friends and family
- More time for yourself
- More intimate time with your partner
- More time for rest and relaxation
- More money because you will no longer purchase things that you do not need
- Less stress because clutter causes chaos and anxiety
- You will live in a cleaner space and it will take less time to clean
- Less waste which is better for the environment
- Less envy
- Your minimalist lifestyle will help you stop comparing your life to others
- More time to follow and pursue your dreams
- You will gain confidence and be able to make decisions quickly.
- Less stuff less to think about. Which shoes? Which purse? Which shirt?
- More time to travel and create experiences
- You will know exactly where everything is

- More freedom, financially, psychologically, mentally, physically, spiritually, and emotionally.
- More money and time? Who doesn't want that?

When you look at the world today and see how prevalent storage spaces have become, and you look at how much people hoard and refuse to part with stuff; it raises a string of questions. The most pressing of which relates to the issue of being able to let go.

For most people the idea of letting go is anathema to them, they detest the idea because it is commonplace to now think that the more you own, the more you can look at your life and think that it is worth more than you feel. It's a two-edged sword. On one side our self-worth is not nearly enough to meet our expectations and so we accumulate things to feel good about ourselves, or we feel that our best days are behind us, therefore, we can't seem to let go. One affects how we think of ourselves in the present and the other affects how we see ourselves in the future. The idea to hold onto things (hoard) is both telling of our current state of mind and the fears we have about our abilities.

It's important that you understand that your best days are ahead of you, especially when you are a minimalist. When you seek and find clarity, everything around you turns into an opportunity. When you ask, you will receive if you are clear.

If you have been asking and asking, repeatedly, but no answer has been forthcoming, don't think that no one is listening. The reason you don't hear an answer to your prayers or wishes is not because there isn't an answer, it is because you do not have the clarity to hear the answer. There is too much going on around you. Imagine asking your boss for a raise while having your ears plugged with your headphones blasting your favorite soundtrack. There's no way for you to hear the answer you are hoping for.

If you want your life to turn around, if you want your life to advance to the next level, if you want to up your game, then you have to clear out all the gunk and junk that's clogging your path. When you clear out your physical gunk and junk, you simultaneously clear out your mental gunk and junk and this automatically results in brighter days ahead.

I'd also like to add that simplifying can be the best gift you can give to your family and loved ones. When you have all of your affairs in order, you will never have to worry about leaving your junk and responsibilities on someone else's shoulders. Too many people lose loved ones, and on top of being sad and grief-stricken, they have to take days and sometimes months to go through the stuff that has been accumulated. They have to decide what to keep, what to sell, and who gets what. I have heard countless stories of those who have lost loved ones who were minimalists and these people are so grateful that they didn't have the burden of having to paw and sort through stuff.

Some people move slowly into the idea of minimalism, and some jump right in and get it done as soon as possible. You didn't pick this book up by accident. If there is something stirring inside of you that is drawing you towards minimalism, then go for it! The key is in the action, though. You can read this book over and over, but if you don't take action, nothing will happen and you won't reach your goals. Make a list of your why's right now, and then take action. Remember to be patient with yourself, but not too patient. You want to see progress. You want to see results, and you will!

ABOUT SAGE WILCOX

Sage lives in the United States with her husband, children, cat, and dog. She is a certified energy healer and is working on becoming a Life Coach. Sage enjoys giving advice to her clients, friends, and family on healing, love, and relationships. She also enjoys studying human behavior, reading, writing, being outdoors, and enhancing her relationships with others. She enjoys reading and learning the Bible. In her experience, the more she learns and practices the Word, the better her life becomes.

Sage is a hopeless romantic! She strives to help others fall madly in love with everything about their lives!

Other books by Sage Wilcox:

- *Love Letters from Exes: Proof That Life Goes On After a Break Up and Love Is What You Make It*
- *Get It Up: 101 Ways to Raise Your Vibration, Reduce Stress, Depression, & Anxiety, Increase Joy, Peace, & Happiness and Attract Abundance Automatically!*
- *The 2-Hour Vacation: Let Go and Relax, Reduce Stress & Anxiety, Gain Inner Peace, and Happiness*
- *Until We Fall (A Romance Novel)*
- *The Importance of Doing It: How to Utilize Discipline to Get Out of Bed, and Make Your Dreams Come True! A Guide to Taking Action to Create Successful Habits, Reduce Stress, Anxiety, & Depression & Gain Self-Discipline, Motivation, & Success!*

Please visit her website at:
http://sagewilcox.wix.com/books

Disclaimer

The purpose of this book is for entertainment purposes only. This book is designed to provide information and motivation to our readers. The content of each article, letter, or insight is the sole expression and opinion of its author, and not necessarily that of the publisher. The letters contained in this book are from contributors and are the contributor's recollections of their experiences. This is a work based on opinions, recollections, and true events, however, names, characters, businesses, places, and incidents are either the products of the authors' imaginations or used in a fictitious manner. Any resemblance to actual persons, living or dead, businesses, companies, events, locales, or actual events is entirely coincidental. This book is not intended nor is it implied to be a substitute for professional medical advice, and any medical advice and any medical information contained in this book is not intended to be diagnostic or treatment in any way. The author and publisher are not engaged in rendering medical, psychological, legal, or any other professional services. If medical, psychological or other expert assistance is required, please talk to your physician and locate the services of a competent professional. The author and publisher shall have neither liability nor responsibility to any person or entity with respect to any loss or damage caused, or alleged to have been caused, directly or indirectly, by the information contained in this book. Neither the publisher nor the individual author(s) shall be liable for any physical, psychological, emotional, financial, or commercial damages, including, but not limited to, special, incidental, consequential or other damages. Our views and rights are the same: You are responsible for your own choices, actions, and results. If you do not wish to be bound by the above, you may return this book along with a copy of the receipt to the publisher for a full refund.

www.ingramcontent.com/pod-product-compliance
Lightning Source LLC
Chambersburg PA
CBHW071620040426
42452CB00009B/1409

9781945290091